Welcome to "Taming Gastritis: A Flavorful Journey to Digestive Wellness Cookbook," where we explore delicious recipes and nutrition tips to help you manage and alleviate the symptoms of gastritis. This cookbook is designed for those who struggle with gastritis, a condition that affects the stomach lining and can cause painful symptoms such as abdominal pain, bloating, and nausea.

Managing gastritis can be a challenging task, but with the right diet and lifestyle modifications, it's possible to reduce symptoms and promote digestive wellness. This cookbook provides a collection of flavorful recipes that are easy to prepare and will help you maintain a healthy diet while also satisfying your taste buds.

In this cookbook, you will find a variety of recipes that are designed to be gentle on the digestive system, including low-fat, low-acid, and low-spice options. We also include recipes that are rich in nutrients that can help alleviate gastritis symptoms and promote overall digestive health. Whether you're looking for breakfast, lunch, or dinner options, we have you covered with a range of delicious recipes.

In addition to the recipes, we also provide nutrition tips and advice on how to manage gastritis through diet and lifestyle modifications. With the help of this cookbook, we hope to provide a flavorful journey towards digestive wellness and make the process of managing gastritis a little easier for you

What is Gastritis?

Gastritis is a medical condition characterized by inflammation, irritation, or erosion of the lining of the stomach. This inflammation is typically caused by various factors, including bacterial infections, long-term use of nonsteroidal anti-inflammatory drugs (NSAIDs), excessive alcohol consumption, stress, and autoimmune diseases. When left untreated, gastritis can lead to severe complications, such as bleeding and stomach ulcers.

There are two types of gastritis: acute and chronic. Acute gastritis is a sudden inflammation of the stomach lining, which can cause symptoms such as stomach pain, nausea, vomiting, and loss of appetite. Chronic gastritis, on the other hand, is a long-term inflammation of the stomach lining that can lead to more serious complications.

Symptoms of Gastritis

The symptoms of gastritis can vary from person to person and can range from mild to severe. Some of the common symptoms of gastritis include:

Abdominal pain or discomfort

Nausea and vomiting

Table of Contents

Introduction...3

What is Gastritis?...4

Symptoms of Gastritis 4

Diagnosis and Treatment..5

Understanding Gastritis...6

Delicious Recipes...9

Conclusion 74

Loss of appetite

Bloating

Belching

Indigestion

Heartburn

Blood in the stool or vomit (in severe cases)

Diagnosis and Treatment

If you experience any of the symptoms of gastritis, it is important to seek medical attention promptly. Your doctor will perform a physical examination and may recommend tests such as an endoscopy, blood test, or stool test to confirm the diagnosis of gastritis.

The treatment for gastritis typically involves a combination of lifestyle changes and medication. For instance, your doctor may recommend that you avoid spicy or acidic foods, alcohol, and tobacco to prevent further irritation of the stomach lining. You may also be prescribed medication such as antacids, proton pump inhibitors, or antibiotics to help relieve the symptoms and treat the underlying cause of the inflammation.

Gastritis is a condition that occurs when the stomach lining becomes inflamed. It can be caused by a variety of factors, including bacterial infections, excessive alcohol consumption, long-term use of nonsteroidal anti-inflammatory drugs (NSAIDs), and stress.

In this chapter, we'll explore the different types of gastritis, their causes, and symptoms. We'll also discuss how to properly diagnose gastritis and work with your healthcare provider to develop a treatment plan.

Types of Gastritis

There are several types of gastritis, each with its own set of causes and symptoms. The most common types include:

Acute gastritis: This type of gastritis occurs suddenly and is often caused by bacterial infections, excessive alcohol consumption, or NSAID use.

Chronic gastritis: Chronic gastritis develops gradually and can last for years. It is often caused by Helicobacter pylori (H. pylori) infections or autoimmune diseases.

Erosive gastritis: This type of gastritis is characterized by erosion of the stomach lining and can be caused by long-term use of NSAIDs or excessive alcohol consumption.

Atrophic gastritis: Atrophic gastritis is a type of chronic gastritis that occurs when the stomach lining thins and loses its function. It is often associated with H. pylori infections or autoimmune diseases.

Causes and Symptoms

The causes of gastritis can vary depending on the type of gastritis, but common causes include bacterial infections, excessive alcohol consumption, long-term use of NSAIDs, and stress.

Symptoms of gastritis can also vary but may include:

Nausea and vomiting

Abdominal pain or discomfort

Loss of appetite

Indigestion or heartburn

Bloating

Belching

Dark or black stools

It's important to note that some people with gastritis may not experience any symptoms at all.

Diagnosis and Treatment

To properly diagnose gastritis, your healthcare provider may perform a physical exam, take a medical history, and order tests such as blood tests, stool tests, or an endoscopy.

Treatment for gastritis depends on the underlying cause and may include medications to reduce inflammation, antibiotics to treat bacterial infections, and lifestyle changes such as avoiding alcohol and NSAIDs.

In this chapter, we'll also discuss natural remedies and dietary changes that can help alleviate symptoms of gastritis and promote digestive wellness

Turkey Sweet Potato Skillet

Ingredients

3 tablespoons olive oil, divided

1 pound 93% lean dark meat ground turkey

1 teaspoon kosher salt, divided

1 teaspoon granulated garlic powder

4 cups chopped sweet potatoes

¼ cup water

TO ADD AT THE END

1 cup packed baby spinach

½ cup Chipotle Honey Vinaigrette, recipe below

⅓ cup grated cheese of choice

FOR THE CHIPOTLE HONEY SAUCE

1 small garlic clove, peeled and finely minced or grated

½ teaspoon kosher salt

2 teaspoons minced chipotle peppers, from a can of chipotles in adobo

2 teaspoons honey, omit for Whole30 or low sugar

1/4 cup fresh lime juice

1/3 cup avocado oil

Freshly ground pepper, to taste

OPTIONAL SERVING SUGGESTIONS

Remaining Chipotle Honey Sauce

Sliced avocado, cilantro, sour cream, cooked rice, cauliflower rice, warm tortillas

Equipment

Skillet

Chef's Knife

Cutting Board

Instructions

In a large, 10" skillet, heat 1 tablespoon olive oil over medium heat. Add the turkey, sprinkle with ½ teaspoon salt and garlic powder, stirring to break into small pieces.

Cook, stirring the ground turkey occasionally, until it's browned and just cooked through, about 5-8 minutes. Remove from the pan and set aside.

While the turkey cooks, prepare the sweet potatoes.

After removing the turkey, and to the same pan, heat 2 tablespoons of olive oil over medium heat. Add the sweet potatoes, sprinkle with ½ teaspoon salt, and stir to combine. Add the water, stirring to scrape any browned bits from the bottom of the pan. Cover, reduce to a simmer, and cook until the sweet potatoes are tender, about 10-15 minutes, stirring occasionally. Add a splash more water if the pan starts to dry out.

While the sweet potatoes cook, make the sauce by whisking together the garlic clove, salt, chipotle peppers, honey, lime juice, avocado oil and pepper in a small bowl, or shaking together in a mason jar.

When the sweet potatoes are cooked, uncover, and add the cooked turkey along with the spinach, and half the Chipotle Honey Sauce until the turkey is warmed through and the spinach is wilted, about 1 minute.

Turn off the heat and sprinkle on the cheese, allowing 2-3 minutes for it to melt.

Taste and add additional sauce if desired. Serve as-is, or with any topping you like.

Chicken Bowls

Ingredients

4 cups sliced cooked Greek Yogurt Chicken Breast, or any cooked chicken

2 cups cooked cauliflower rice, or any cooked grain such as couscous, quinoa, or rice

1 cup chopped English or Persian cucumber

1 cup halved cherry tomatoes

1 cup sliced red or orange bell pepper

¼ cup thinly sliced red onion

¼ cup kalamata olives

¼ cup crumbled feta cheese

½ cup Yogurt Tahini Dressing

OPTIONAL SERVING SUGGESTIONS

freshly squeezed lemon juice

flat leaf parsley

toasted pita

Equipment

Chef's Knife

Cutting Board

Instructions

Divide the cauliflower rice or grain between four bowls. Top each with the cooked chicken, cucumber, tomatoes, bell pepper, red onion, olive, and feta. Drizzle with the Yogurt Tahini Dressing and serve.

Skillet Chicken and Sweet Potatoes

Ingredients

1 pound chicken thighs, about 4 chicken thighs, or boneless, skinless chicken breast cut into large pieces

1 teaspoon salt, divided

1 ½ pounds sweet potatoes, cut into ½ inch pieces

2 tablespoons avocado oil, divided (or other neutral flavored oil)

2 tablespoons butter, or plant-based butter for dairy-free

2 tablespoons honey

1 teaspoon chipotle, from a can of chipotle peppers in adobo, minced

1 garlic clove, minced or finely grated

Equipment

Skillet

Chef's Knife

Cutting Board

Instructions

Preheat the oven to 350F.

Sprinkle the chicken on both sides with ½ teaspoon salt.

Heat 1 tablespoon of avocado oil in a large, 12-inch skillet over medium-high heat.

Add the chicken and allow it to brown 3-4 minutes one one side. Flip and cook for an additional 3-4 minutes, or until browned. Remove to a plate and set aside.

Turn the heat down to medium, add the remaining 1 tablespoon avocado oil along with the sweet potatoes. Sprinkle with ½ teaspoon salt, and cook for 5 minutes, stirring frequently.

Meanwhile, melt the butter, honey, chipotle, and garlic together, either in the microwave or on the stovetop.

When the potatoes are slightly browned, add back the chicken along with any accumulated juices. Pour over the honey and butter mixture, stirring to combine.

Place in the oven and bake for 10-15 minutes, or until the chicken is cooked through and no longer pink in the middle.

Chicken Zucchini Skillet

Ingredients

2 tbsp olive oil, divided

1 lb boneless, skinless chicken breasts or thighs, cut into 1 inch pieces

1 tsp no-salt added Italian seasoning

1 tsp kosher salt, divided

4 cups 1-inch diced zucchini , (from about 4 medium zucchini)

2 garlic cloves, finely minced or grated

1 15-oz can diced tomatoes

1 tbsp tomato paste

1/2 cup chicken stock

2 tbsp butter*

1/4 cup lightly packed fresh basil, thinly sliced

 red pepper flakes to taste

Equipment

Skillet

Chef's Knife

Cutting Board

Instructions

In a large 12-inch skillet, heat 1 tablespoon olive oil over medium high heat. Add the chicken in one layer, taking care not to overlap the pieces. Sprinkle with the Italian seasoning and ½ teaspoon salt.

Cook the chicken undisturbed, until golden brown on one side, about 5 minutes. Flip, and cook an additional 3 minutes until browned on both sides and just cooked through. Remove from the pan and set aside.

In the same pan, heat the remaining 1 tablespoon olive oil over medium heat. Add the zucchini, sprinkle with ½ teaspoon salt, and cook until just tender, stirring occasionally, about 5 minutes.

Add the garlic, and cook until fragrant, about 1 minutes, stirring occasionally.

Add chicken stock, stirring to deglaze, then add tomato paste and diced tomatoes, stirring until well combined.

Add the cooked chicken back to the pan, turn the heat to medium low, and simmer uncovered for 5 minutes, until the sauce is slightly reduced.

Turn off the heat, add the butter, and stir to combine. Taste the sauce and add additional salt if desired. Serve sprinkled with basil and red pepper flakes to taste.

Honey Orange Dijon Chicken Skewers

Ingredients

FOR THE HONEY ORANGE DIJON SAUCE

3 tbsp Dijon mustard

2 tbsp honey, (omit for Whole30)

1/4 cup fresh squeezed orange juice , (from about 1 medium orange)

1/4 cup olive oil

1/2 tsp kosher salt

1/4 tsp freshly ground pepper

1 tbsp minced fresh sage

FOR THE HONEY ORANGE DIJON CHICKEN SKEWERS

6 10-inch bamboo skewers , presoaked

2 lbs boneless, skinless chicken thighs, excess fat trimmed, and cut into 1-inch chunks

Equipment

Chef's Knife

Cutting Board

Instructions

In a medium bowl or mason jar, combine the mustard, honey, orange juice, olive oil, salt, pepper and sage, whisking or shaking until well combined.

Place the cubed chicken in a bowl. Add half the sauce and marinade for at least an hour, or all day in the refrigerator, covered.

Remove the chicken from the marinade, shaking off any excess. Thread onto bamboo skewers. Discard extra marinade.

Preheat the grill to medium-high heat (about 400F). When the grill is hot, place the skewers on the grill and cook for 7-8 minutes, flipping halfway, until the chicken is cooked through and grill marks have formed.

Serve with remaining sauce, atop rice, and slaw if you prefer.

Pot Turmeric Chicken Soup

Ingredients

3 tablespoons olive oil

1 cup chopped yellow onion

2 cups chopped carrot

2 cups chopped celery

1 tablespoon turmeric

¼ teaspoon ground pepper

2 teaspoons kosher salt, divided

2 pounds boneless skinless chicken breasts or thighs

1 quart chicken stock

1 cup water

Equipment

Instant Pot

Slow Cooker

Cutting Board

Chef's Knife

Instructions

INSTANT POT INSTRUCTIONS

Add the olive oil to an electric pressure cooker. Turn to saute, add the onion and ¼ teaspoon salt and saute for 4 minutes.

Add the carrots, celery, ¼ teaspoon salt, turmeric and pepper, stirring to combine.

Salt the chicken on both sides using ¼ teaspoon salt. Add the chicken in a single layer on top of the vegetables.

Pour in the chicken stock, water, and remaining 1 ½ teaspoon salt.

Secure the lid, select the manual setting, and set it to high pressure for 15 minutes. Your instant pot may take anywhere from 25-35+ minutes to come to pressure before the cook time starts.

When the pressure cooker timer is done, quick release the pressure.

Remove the chicken, and shred or chop into bite sized pieces. Add back to the pressure cooker, stirring to combine. Taste, adding additional salt or pepper if desired.

SLOW COOKER INSTRUCTIONS

Add the olive oil to a medium pan over medium heat. Add the onion and ¼ teaspoon salt, cooking until soft, stirring occasionally, about 5 minutes.

Add the carrots, celery, ¼ teaspoon salt, turmeric and pepper, stirring to combine.

Add the vegetable mixture to a 6-quart slow cooker.

Salt the chicken on both sides using ¼ teaspoon salt. Add the chicken in a single layer on top of the vegetables.

Pour in the chicken stock, water, and remaining 1 ½ teaspoon salt.

Cover and cook on high for 4 hours, or low for 6, or until the chicken is cooked through and the vegetables are tender.

Remove the chicken, and shred or chop into bite sized pieces. Add back to the slow cooker, stirring to combine. Taste, adding additional salt or pepper if desired.

Waist-friendly Waldorf salad

Ingredients:

4 large apples (use a combination of red delicious and granny smith), cored and cubed

4 stalks celery, chopped

1 cup chopped walnuts

½ cup raisins

2 tablespoons walnut oil

1 tablespoon apple cider vinegar

salt and pepper to taste

Instructions:

Toss together the apples, celery, walnuts, and raisins. In a small bowl, whisk the walnut oil with the apple cider vinegar and seasonings. Pour over the salad, combine, and serve over a bed of greens.

Sautéed Mackerel

Ingredients:

two, 1/2 pound mackerel fillets

salt and pepper

2 tablespoons olive oil

lemon juice

Heat a sauté pan over high heat and add the olive oil. Season the fillets and place them into the pan. Cook for three to five minutes. Flip and cook the other side until golden brown on the outside and flaky-white in the center. Top with a squeeze of lemon.

Milk soup with pumpkin

Ingredients:

1 cup of water

300 g of pumpkin

2 tbsp of semolina

3 cups of milk

1 tbsp of butter

2 tsp of sugar

salt to taste

How to cook:

Pour a thin stream of semolina in the boiling milk. Cook it for about 15 minutes.

Cut pumpkin into pieces, boil in a little water, and smash it with broth.

Add the pumpkin in a saucepan, bring the soup to a boil. Season with salt, add sugar.

Potato and carrot puree

Ingredients:

4-5 potatoes

2 carrots

2 tbsp of butter

1 cup of milk

How to cook:

Peel and then boil potatoes and carrots. Add salt.

Drain the broth. Smash vegetables with blender.

Add warmed milk, butter, and whip it up.

Pate with lean meat

Ingredients:

500 grams of lean meat of rabbit or veal

200 g of chicken liver

2 tbsp of vegetable oil

1/3 of white loaf

parsley to taste

3-4 carrots

1/3 cup of milk

1 egg

butter to taste

salt to taste

How to cook:

Cut meat and liver into pieces, cover with cold water and boil on low heat.

Peel carrot and add it to the meat cooking (it can be cut into large chunks).

Soak bread in water with milk.

Make mince from meat and liver, add a sodden bread without crusts.

Add the egg, parsley, salt and mince. Mix everything together.

Bake the mass of pate, greased with oil, in the oven, for 30-40 minutes.

Potato Soup

Ingredients

2 small sweet potatoes

1 cup vegetable broth

1 carrot

1 avocado

1 cup spinach

Salt to taste

Directions

Wash and peel potatoes. Chop into cubes and press.

Wash, cut and press carrot.

Slice avocado in half. Remove the pit and scoop the flesh out. Mix with broth and press

Transfer about ½ of the pulp into pot. Add squeezed juice and a pinch of salt. On medium heat bring to a boil. Stir until everything is nicely combined.

Wash and press spinach. Combine spinach juice and pulp, stir until smooth, and warm it lightly. Pour into the middle of each soup and serve.

Matcha Protein Shake

Ingredients

1 frozen banana, broken into chunks

2 teaspoons matcha powder

1 cup packed baby spinach

1 tablespoon ground flax seed

1 cup unsweetened milk of choice

2 scoops vanilla protein powder , plant-based protein powder for vegan

optional: ice

Equipment

Blender

Cutting Board

Chef's Knife

Instructions

Add all the ingredients to a high speed blender. Blend on high until smooth.

Protein Chia Pudding

Ingredients

2 tablespoons chia seeds

½ cup plus 2 tablespoons unsweetened almond milk, or milk of choice

1 scoop protein powder , of choice

2 teaspoons liquid sweetener of choice such as maple syrup or honey, (optional)

SUGGESTED TOPPINGS

1 tablespoon nut or seed butter, fresh strawberries, fresh blueberries

Equipment

Mason Jar

Instructions

To an 8-ounce wide mason jar, or other jar with tightly fitting lid, add 2 tablespoons chia seeds and one scoop of protein powder, stirring with a fork to combine.

Add the milk and sweetener, if using. Secure the lid, then shake vigorously until all the ingredients have combined and protein powder dissolves.

Allow to sit for 5 minutes, then shake vigorously again.

Allow to sit an additional 5 minutes, shake vigorously, then refrigerate for at least 3 hours or up to 5 days, covered.

Serve chilled or at room temperature, with nut butter and fresh berries if desired.

Pumpkin Spice Protein Shake

Ingredients

1 cup frozen riced cauliflower

¾ cup pumpkin puree

⅓ cup unsweetened greek yogurt

1 tablespoon almond butter

1 teaspoon pumpkin pie spice

1 serving vanilla protein powder, (or pumpkin spice protein powder)

3/4 cup unsweetened almond milk, (or milk of choice)

OPTIONAL TOPPINGS

whipped cream or coconut cream

pumpkin pie spice

Equipment

Blender

Instructions

Add all the ingredients to a high speed blender. Blend until smooth.

Green Protein Smoothie

Ingredients

1 frozen banana

2 cups baby spinach

1 tablespoon chia seeds

1 cup unsweetened milk of choice, such as almond or cashew milk

1 scoop vanilla protein powder

1 tablespoon peanut butter

Equipment

High Speed Blender

Instructions

Add all the ingredients to a high speed blender. Blend on high until smooth.

Golden Glow Turmeric Flourless Muffins

Ingredients

⅓ cup melted coconut oil, plus more for greasing the pan

2 large eggs

⅔ cup unsweetened applesauce

⅓ cup pure maple syrup

1 teaspoon vanilla extract

2 ⅓ cups almond or oat flour*

½ teaspoon baking soda

½ teaspoon baking powder

¼ teaspoon kosher salt

2 teaspoons ground turmeric

½ teaspoon cinnamon

½ teaspoon ground ginger

⅛ teaspoon freshly ground pepper**

⅓ cup dairy-free chocolate chips, plus more for sprinkling

Equipment

Muffin Tin

Instructions

Heat the oven to 350F.

In a large bowl, whisk together the coconut oil, eggs, applesauce, maple syrup, and vanilla extract.

Add the flour, baking soda, baking powder, salt, turmeric, cinnamon, ginger, and pepper. Stir until well incorporated.

Add the chocolate chips, stirring to combine.

Fill each section of a greased, 12-section muffin tin with roughly ¼ cup batter. Sprinkle the tops with chocolate chips, then bake for 15-20 minutes, or until the edges begin to pull away from the sides and a toothpick comes out clean.

Allow to cool in the pan for 5 minutes, then cool the rest on a cooling rack.

Berry Protein Smoothie

Ingredients

1 cup frozen mixed berries , (or any combination of strawberries, raspberries, blueberries and blackberries)

1 tbsp chia seeds

1 tbsp unsweetened almond butter , (or nut butter of choice or use seed butter for nut-free)

2 tbsp vanilla protein powder

1 tbsp fresh lemon juice

1 cup unsweetened almond milk , (or milk of choice)

Equipment

Blender

Instructions

Add all the ingredients to a high speed blender. Blend on high until well smooth. Serve immediately.

Sweet Potato Hashbrown Egg Nests

Ingredients

2 medium russet potatoes, scrubbed clean

2 medium sweet potatoes, scrubbed clean

3 tablespoons olive oil, plus more for greasing the muffin tin

¼ teaspoon kosher salt, plus more for sprinkling

12 large eggs

Equipment

Box Grater

Muffin Tin

Instructions

Preheat the oven to 400 degrees.

Bake the russet and sweet potatoes until they're cooked through but not quite tender, about 20 minutes. The goal is just to pre-bake them a bit, so they should still be pretty firm.

Let the potatoes cool enough to handle, then peel and grate, using the largest grating size.

In a large bowl, toss the grated potatoes, olive oil, and salt.

Grease the muffin tin with olive oil.

Add the grated potato mixture to a 12-cup muffin pan, 1/3 cup at a time. The mixture will shrink significantly when baked, so it's okay if there's a lot of mixture in each cup. If you end up with extra potato mixture, feel free to use it to make additional egg cups.

Use your fingers to lightly press the center of each cup so the potatoes spill over the top a bit.

Increase the oven temperature to 425 degrees, then bake until the potatoes are golden brown, about 20-25 minutes. Keep on eye on them so the ends of the potato shreds don't burn.

Remove from the oven, let the nests cool a bit, then crack one egg into each cup and sprinkle with additional kosher salt to taste.

Return to the oven and bake for 10-15 minutes, depending on how cooked you like your eggs. Let cool slightly, then serve immediately.

Kale and Sweet Potato Egg Cups

Ingredients

2 tablespoons olive oil

1 bunch Lacinato, Dinosaur kale, stems removed and very thinly sliced (about 2 cups)

1 large sweet potato, grated (about 2 cups)

½ teaspoon salt, divided

12 large eggs

Instructions

Preheat the oven to 350 degrees.

Heat the olive oil over medium heat in a large pan. Add the kale and cook for 5 minutes, stirring occasionally.

Add the sweet potatoes, sprinkle with ¼ teaspoon salt, and cook for 10 minutes, or until the sweet potatoes are softened, stirring occasionally. Set aside and allow to cool. They may stick a bit, so just do your best to scrape the bits from the bottom of the pan.

In a large bowl, whisk together the eggs and ¼ teaspoon salt. Add the cooked, cooled sweet potato and kale mixture, stirring until well combined.

Pour the egg mixture into a 12-cup muffin tin (I like to use silicone liners to avoid sticking), dividing the mixture evenly between the cups. The mixture should come to near the top of each cup.

Bake for 20-25 minutes, or until puffed and cooked through.

Remove from the oven and allow to cool. Serve warm or refrigerate in a tightly sealed container for up to 4 days.

Alternatively, place the cooled cups on a baking sheet in the freezer. Allow to freeze completely, then place in a zip-top bag or tightly sealed container for up to a month.

Black Bean Salad with Corn

Ingredients

1 15-oz can black beans, drained and rinsed

1 cup corn kernels , (fresh or frozen)

1 cup halved cherry tomatoes

1 cup chopped bell pepper, red, yellow, or orange

2 tbsp diced red onion

1/2 cup chopped cilantro

CUMIN LIME DRESSING

2 tbsp fresh lime juice , (from 2 limes)

2 tbsp apple cider vinegar

½ tsp plus ⅛ teaspoon kosher salt

½ tsp cumin

½ tsp granulated garlic powder

⅓ cup olive oil

Equipment

Chef's Knife

Cutting Board

Instructions

In a large bowl, mix together the black beans, corn kernels, cherry tomatoes, bell pepper, red onion, and cilantro until well combined. Set aside.

Make the dressing by adding the lime juice, apple cider vinegar, salt, cumin, garlic powder, and olive oil in a small mason jar. Shake until well combined. Alternatively, add the ingredients to a small bowl and whisk to combine.

Pour the dressing over the black bean mixture, stirring to combine. Allow to sit for 5 minutes, then taste for seasoning, adding additional lime juice or salt to taste. Serve at room temperature or store (covered) in the refrigerator for up to 5 days.

Curry Quinoa Salad

Ingredients

2 cups dry quinoa

1 (15-oz) can chickpeas, drained and rinsed

2 tablespoons mild curry powder

½ cup extra virgin olive oil

¼ cup apple cider vinegar

2 teaspoons kosher salt, divided

1 lemon, zested and juiced

2 small cloves garlic, minced

2 cups English cucumber, diced, from about 1 large

2 cups diced green apple, from about 2 medium

2 cups diced red bell peppers, from about 2 large

¼ cup packed basil leaves, thinly sliced

1/3 cup roasted and salted sunflower seeds

Instructions

Rinse the quinoa. Combine rinsed quinoa with the curry powder, 1 teaspoon salt, and 4 cups cold water in a large pot. Cover, bring to a boil, then reduce heat to low and simmer, covered, for 18 minutes. Turn the heat off and let sit, covered, an additional 5 minutes.

In a large bowl make the dressing by combining the olive oil, vinegar, 1 teaspoon salt, lemon juice, lemon zest, and garlic, whisking until well combined.

To the dressing add the chickpeas, cucumber, apple, and peppers. Add the warm quinoa and stir until well combined. The mixture will be on the wet side. Let sit at least an hour for the dressing to absorb and flavors to develop.

Stir in the basil and half the sunflower seeds then cover and chill for up to 3 days. When ready to serve bring to room temperature and serve with a sprinkling of the remaining sunflower seeds.

Lentil Salad

Ingredients

2 cups dry brown lentils, rinsed and picked through

1 tablespoon olive oil

¼ teaspoon kosher salt

4 cups diced butternut squash

2 cups microgreens or baby sprouts

¼ cup roasted pumpkin seeds

FOR THE DRESSING

¼ cup red wine vinegar

1 garlic clove, minced

1 tablespoon pure maple syrup

1 teaspoon dijon mustard

½ teaspoon salt

⅓ cup extra virgin olive oil

Optional toppings: Sliced avocado, feta cheese, fresh figs

Instructions

Preheat the oven to 400F.

Add the lentils to a medium saucepan and cover with at least four inches of water. Cover, bring to a boil, then reduce to low and simmer for 15-25 minutes, or until the lentils are just tender but not mushy. Cooking times vary depending on the type and freshness of lentils used, so start testing at 15 minutes. Drain and set aside.

Meanwhile, add the butternut squash to a rimmed baking sheet, drizzle with 1 tablespoon olive oil, and sprinkle with ¼ teaspoon salt.

Place in the oven and roast for 20-25 minutes, flipping halfway through, or until the squash is golden brown on each side and cooked through.

Make the dressing by whisking the vinegar, garlic, maple syrup, mustard, and salt in a medium bowl. Drizzle in the olive oil and whisk until the dressing is smooth and well combined.

Combine the warm, drained lentils with the dressing in a large bowl, tossing to combine. Let sit for 5 minutes for the dressing to absorb.

Add the roasted squash, microgreens, and pumpkin seeds tossing to combine. Serve immediately, or store, tightly sealed in the fridge for up to 5 days.

Quinoa Bowl

Ingredients

FOR THE BOWLS

1 cup quinoa, rinsed and drained

½ teaspoon salt

1 15- oz can chickpeas, or 2 cup cooked lentils or white beans

1 English cucumber, thinly sliced

1-2 bell peppers, red, orange, or yellow, thinly sliced

1 pint cherry tomatoes

4 cups baby spinach

FOR THE TAHINI DRESSING

¼ cup tahini, sesame seed paste

1 clove garlic, very finely minced or grated

½ cup red wine vinegar

¼ teaspoon salt

¼ teaspoon dried oregano

1 teaspoon honey

⅓ cup warm water

Instructions

Place the rinsed, drained quinoa in a medium saucepan. Add 2 cups of water and the salt. Cover, bring to a boil, then reduce to a simmer. Simmer, covered, for 18 minutes. Turn off the heat and let sit for an additional 5 minutes. Uncover and fluff with a fork.

Add the rinsed, drained chickpeas and stir to warm through.

In a medium bowl or jar, whisk or shake together the tahini, garlic, vinegar, salt, oregano, honey and water until very well combined.

Assemble by dividing the spinach, quinoa/chickpea mixture, cucumber, bell peppers, and tomatoes in bowls. Drizzle with the Tahini Dressing and serve.

Golden Glow Chicken Salad

Ingredients

¼ cup fresh lemon juice

1 tablespoon apple cider vinegar

1 teaspoon Dijon mustard

2 teaspoons honey, omit for whole30

2 teaspoons mild curry powder

1 teaspoon salt

⅓ cup extra virgin olive oil

FOR THE SALAD

2 cups cooked diced protein, e.g., chicken, hard boiled egg, canned + drained tuna, chickpeas

1 cup diced English cucumber

1 cup diced green apple

1 cup diced red bell peppers

2 tablespoons chopped green onion

¼ cup roasted, salted sunflower seeds

Instructions

Make the dressing by whisking together the lemon juice, apple cider vinegar, mustard, honey, curry powder and salt in a small bowl. Drizzle in the olive oil and whisk until well combined.

Make the salad by combining the protein, cucumber, apple, bell pepper, and green onion in a large bowl. Add the dressing and toss to coat.

Allow to sit for 5-10 minutes for the flavors to absorb.

Serve and enjoy immediately, topped with sunflower seeds, or cover and store for up to 5 days, with sunflowers seeds as a topping.

Veggie Quinoa Power Bowls

Ingredients

THE LEMON DRESSING

¼ cup freshly squeezed lemon juice, from about 2-3 lemons

¼-½ teaspoon kosher salt

1 teaspoon raw honey

⅓ cup extra virgin olive oil

2 scallions, white and green part, finely chopped

THE VEGGIES

2 medium zucchini, sliced lengthwise

2 medium yellow squash, sliced lengthwise

2 red bell peppers, seeds and stem removed, sliced into large pieces

1 large red onion, cut into 4-5 slices

THE BOWLS

3 cups cooked quinoa

2 cups arugula or baby spinach

1 cup cherry tomatoes, halved

1 cup homemade or prepared hummus

Instructions

In a small bowl, whisk together the lemon juice, salt, and honey. Stream in the olive oil and whisk until well combined. Add the scallions and stir.

Place the veggies (zucchini, yellow squash, bell peppers, and red onion) in a large rimmed pan or baking dish. Pour over ¼ cup of the dressing, tossing to coat. Reserve the remaining dressing for the bowls.

Heat an outdoor grill or grill pan to medium heat. Grill the veggies for 5 minutes, flip, then grill an additional 4-5 minutes until golden and just cooked through. Remove to a pan and set aside.

Assemble by dividing the quinoa evenly between 4 bowls. Top each with the grilled veggies, arugula, cherry tomatoes, and hummus. Drizzle each with the remaining dressing, and serve.

Chicken Apple Salad

Ingredients

FOR THE VINAIGRETTE

1 tablespoon whole grain mustard

1 teaspoon honey, optional

½ teaspoon salt

3 tablespoons white wine vinegar

4 tablespoons extra virgin olive oil

1 small shallot, very thinly sliced

FOR THE CHICKEN SALAD

2 cups chopped apple, from about 2 medium apples

2 cups chopped celery, from about 8-10 stalks

2 cups chopped cooked chicken breasts or thighs, from Garlic Rosemary Roasted Chicken or store-bought rotisserie

⅓ cup chopped roasted, salted cashews

4 cups arugula or spinach, optional

Equipment

Chef's Knife

Cutting Board

Instructions

In a large bowl, whisk together the mustard, honey, salt, vinegar, and olive oil until well combined.

Add the shallot, stir and allow to sit for 5 minutes.

Add the apple, celery, cooked chicken, and cashews, stirring until well combined.

Serve over greens if you like.

Sweet Pea Power Salad

Ingredients

FOR THE SALAD

1 15- oz can chickpeas, rinsed, drained, and patted dried

1 large sweet potato, scrubbed and chopped into 1-inch pieces

2 tablespoons olive oil, divided

½ teaspoon salt, divided

1 4- oz box OrganicGirl Sweet Pea greens mix

FOR THE PEA PESTO DRESSING

½ cup frozen peas, defrosted (fresh peas will also work)

1 clove garlic, minced or grated

⅓ cup raw sunflower seeds

3 tablespoons nutritional yeast

¼ cup freshly squeezed lemon juice, from about 1 large lemon

½ teaspoon salt

⅓ cup extra virgin olive oil

Instructions

Heat the oven to 400 degrees Fahrenheit

Place the chickpeas on a baking sheet, drizzle with 1 tablespoon olive oil and ¼ teaspoon salt. Roast for 25 minutes, stirring once. Remove from the oven and allow to cool.

Place the sweet potatoes on a baking sheet, drizzle with 1 tablespoon olive oil and ¼ teaspoon salt. Roast for 30 minutes, or until lightly browned and tender, flipping halfway through. Remove from the oven and allow to cool. (The chickpeas and the sweet potatoes can roast in the same oven, at the same time, just Wuse different racks).

While the chickpeas and sweet potatoes roast, make the dressing by combining the peas, garlic, sunflower seeds, nutritional yeast, lemon juice, and ½ teaspoons salt in a food processor. Pulse until the ingredients are well combined. Turn to high and drizzle in the olive oil. Continue to blend until the dressing is thick and creamy.

Assemble the salad by placing a handful of greens on a plate. Sprinkle with roasted sweet potatoes, chickpeas, and drizzle generously with the Pea Pesto Dressing. Serve immediately.

Turmeric Tahini Loaded Chicken Salad

Ingredients

FOR THE TURMERIC TAHINI DRESSING

1 teaspoon turmeric

1 tablespoon tahini, sesame seed butter

1 garlic clove, minced or finely grated

1 teaspoon honey, omit for Whole30

¼ teaspoon kosher salt

2 tablespoons apple cider vinegar

⅓ cup extra virgin olive oil

FOR THE SALAD

2 cups cooked shredded chicken*

1 cup shredded carrots

1 cup slaw mix or finely shredded cabbage

1-2 green onion, finely chopped

¼ cup sulfite-free raisins

Equipment

Chef's Knife

Cutting Board

Instructions

In a medium bowl, add the turmeric, tahini, garlic, honey (if using), salt, pepper, and vinegar, stirring to combine. Drizzle in the olive oil and whisk until smooth. Alternatively, add all the ingredients to a blender and blend until smooth.

In a large bowl, add the chicken, carrots, slaw or cabbage, green onions, and raisins. Add the dressing, stirring to combine. Allow to sit for 15 minutes for the flavors to combine.

Serve over greens, if desired.

Crockpot White Chicken Chili

Ingredients

1 ½ pounds boneless skinless chicken breasts, or thighs

1 onion, finely chopped

2 (15-oz) cans white beans, drained and rinsed (such as Great Northern or cannellini)

1 (4.5-oz) can mild diced green chilis

1 cup mild green salsa verde , tomatillo salsa

1 cup chicken stock

1 teaspoon granulated garlic powder

1 teaspoon ground cumin

½-1 teaspoon kosher salt

TO ADD AT THE END

4 tablespoons cream cheese, traditional or dairy free

OPTIONAL TOPPINGS

Avocado, sour cream (traditional or dairy-free), crushed tortilla chips, chopped onion, cilantro, fresh lime juice, jalapeno, Monterey jack cheese or dairy-free cheese shreds

Equipment

Slow Cooker

Immersion Blender

Chef's Knife

Cutting Board

Instructions

SLOW COOKER INSTRUCTIONS

Add the chicken, onion, white beans, green chilis, salsa verde, chicken stock, garlic powder, cumin, and salt to a 6-quart slow cooker.

Cover and cook on high for 4-5 hours or low for 6-8 hours.

Uncover, remove the chicken, and shred with two forks or dice into chunks.

Using an immersion blender, blend the bean mixture for 5-10 seconds. Alternatively, carefully, remove ½ to 1 cup of the bean mixture to a blender. Cover, blend on high, then add back to the chili, stirring to combine. Note: Blending for just a few seconds will add a creaminess to the chili, while leaving the texture of most of the beans.

Ladle a few tablespoons of the bean mixture into a medium bowl. Add the cream cheese and stir until well incorporated.

Add the chicken back to the slow cooker, along with the bean-puree-cream-cheese mixture, stirring to combine. Taste and add additional salt or salsa if desired.

Serve with any toppings you like.

Chicken Vegetable Soup

Ingredients

1 tablespoon olive oil

1 medium onion, chopped

1 cup chopped carrot, about 1 large

½ cup chopped celery, about 2 stalks

2 tablespoons tomato paste

1 teaspoon granulated garlic powder

1 ½ teaspoon kosher salt, divided

2 cups peeled, chopped Russet potatoes (about 1 large)

1 15- oz can diced tomatoes, with juices

1 bay leaf

1 quart chicken stock

1 ½ pounds boneless skinless chicken tenders, or boneless skinless chicken breasts sliced into strips, or boneless skinless chicken thighs sliced into strips, or 2 cups shredded cooked rotisserie chicken

TO ADD AT THE END:

2 cups chopped green beans, fresh or frozen, defrosted

1 cup corn kernels, fresh or frozen, defrosted

1 cup peas, fresh or frozen, defrosted

OPTIONAL SERVING SUGGESTIONS:

Fresh basil, fresh parsley, parmesan cheese, red pepper flakes, extra virgin olive oil for drizzling, crusty bread

Equipment

Dutch Oven

Cutting Board

Chef's Knife

Instructions

STOVETOP INSTRUCTIONS

To a large pot or Dutch oven, heat the olive oil over medium heat. Add the onion, sprinkle with ¼ teaspoon salt, and cook, stirring occasionally, until it begins to soften, about 3 minutes.

Add the carrot and celery, stirring to combine. Sprinkle with ¼ teaspoon salt and the garlic powder, then cook for an additional 3-5 minutes until slightly softened, stirring occasionally.

Add the tomato paste, stirring until fragrant, about 1 minute.

Add the potatoes, diced tomatoes, bay leaf, remaining 1 teaspoon salt and chicken, stirring to combine.

Add the stock, cover, bring to a boil, then reduce to a simmer. Cook, covered, for 15-25 minutes until the potatoes are tender and the chicken is cooked through.

Uncover and remove the chicken to a cutting board. Add the green beans to the pot, and stir.

Shred chicken with two forks, or chop into bite-sized pieces.

Turn off the heat, then add back the chicken, along with adding the corn and peas, stirring to combine. Taste and add additional salt if desired.

Golden Gut Healing Soup

INGREDIENTS

4 cups chicken bone broth no salt or low sodium

3 carrots peeled

1 celery

1 1/2 cup sugar snap peas

1 cup cooked chicken pulled

1 cup spinach

1 tbsp tumeric

salt and pepper to taste

INSTRUCTIONS

Put broth in a medium sauce pan and bring to a boil.

While broth is heating prep your veggies. Chop carrots and celery into 1/4 in slices. Cut snap peas in half at an angle, because we fancy.

Once broth is boiling add carrots and celery, cooking for 3 minutes. Add snap peas and turmeric and bring pot down to a simmer.

Simmer 15 minutes.

Pull off heat and mix in spinach. Once wilted add chicken and serve!

Ginger & Turmeric Carrot Soup

ingredients

Olive oil

Leek

Fennel – This recipe uses fresh fennel, not fennel seeds.

Carrots

Butternut squash – You can use other types of squash, but butternut is definitely preferable.

Garlic

Ginger – You'll need to grate the ginger.

Turmeric powder

Salt

Pepper

Vegetable broth – I like to use a low-sodium veggie broth.

Coconut milk – Lite coconut milk is my preference for this recipe, rather than full-fat coconut milk.

instructions

This soup takes less than an hour to make, but tastes like it's been simmering away on your stove all day long. Here's how to make it.

Cook the veggies. Heat the olive oil in a large pan or dutch oven. Add the carrots, squash, fennel, and leeks, and sauté until the veggies start to soften. This should take 3-5 minutes. Then add the ginger, garlic, turmeric, salt, and pepper, and sauté for 2-3 more minutes.

Add the liquid. Pour in the vegetable broth and coconut milk. Bring the soup to a boil, then lower the temperature, cover, and simmer for 20 minutes.

Blend. Add the soup to a blender, and blend until it is smooth and creamy.

Season. Taste the soup and adjust the seasonings as necessary. Then serve!

Watermelon Pineapple Smoothie

Ingredients

1 frozen banana

1 cup fresh pineapple

1/2 cup 2% or nonfat plain greek yogurt

1/4 cup unsweetened almond milk, plus more if necessary

1/2 teaspoons fresh grated ginger or 1/4 tsp ground ginger

1/2 teaspoons ground turmeric

2 teaspoons of chia seeds

Optional: A few fresh mint leaves

Instructions

Place all ingredients in a blender and mix until smooth. Pour into 2 glasses and enjoy immediately. Makes 2 smoothies.

Tomato free pasta sause

INGREDIENTS

3 medium celery stalks

3 medium carrots, peeled

2 medium zucchinis

1 medium beet

1/2 a small-medium turnip, peeled

2 cups of bone or vegetable broth (or more as needed)

7–10 fresh basil leaves

3–4 tbsp of grapeseed oil or extra virgin olive oil

1 tsp each of garlic powder and onion powder (omit if unable to tolerate)

1/2 teaspoon of dried oregano

1 tsp of salt to add to sauce, plus a little more to season vegetables while cooking

pepper to taste

INSTRUCTIONS

Preheat oven to 400 degrees F.

Prep vegetables: Peel the carrots and turnip. Cut the leafy tops close to the top of the beet, and trim the ends off of the zucchini, celery, carrots and turnip. Cut vegetables (except beet) into two-inch chunks. Since we will only be using half of the turnip in this recipe, you can either cook all of the turnip or set the raw half that won't be used aside for use in other meals. Another option is doubling the recipe. Don't bother peeling the beet, as the skin is very tough to peel when raw. Peel it once it is cooked and slightly cooled.

Spread the cut up zucchini, carrots, celery, turnip and out onto a large rimmed baking sheet lined with parchment paper. Drizzle with 2-3 tbsps of grapeseed or olive oil and sprinkle with desired amount of salt and pepper, then cover using parchment paper, tucking it snugly underneath.

Wash the beet using a vegetable brush, then pat dry. Place in a baking dish lined with parchment paper and drizzle with 1 tbsp of olive oil. Cover using parchment paper, tucking the ends underneath.

Place vegetables in preheated oven and cook until they are tender and can be easily pierced with a fork. Stir the carrots, zucchini, celery, and turnip occasionally while cooking.

Once the beet is done cooking, let it cool slightly. Once cool, submerge it in a bowl of cold water and peel off the outer layer. Cut it in half and place that half in a high-speed blender or food processor. Feel free to add more if you want a deeper red color (keep in mind this will add a more earthy flavor to the sauce). Save the leftover beet for salads or other meals.

Add the remaining cooked vegetables, broth, and fresh basil to the blender. Process until you have a smooth consistency. Add the blended liquid to a saucepan along with the oregano, garlic powder, onion powder, salt, and pepper. Cook on medium-low for 4-5 minutes while stirring. Add more broth as needed for a thinner consistency.

Remove from heat and serve with pasta or use as tomato/marinara sauce replacement.

Baked Chicken

INGREDIENTS

1 tsp Each of Cumin, Basil, Oregano, and Parsley

1/2 tsp Each of Thyme, Rosemary, and Turmeric

1/4 tsp Red Pepper and Ginger

1 pound Chicken Breast, cut into strips

1 Tbsp Butter

1 Tbsp Olive Oil

1/4 cup Rice Chex, crushed

INSTRUCTIONS

Preheat oven to 400 F.

In a small bowl, mix together all spices.

Melt butter and mix with olive oil.

Place chicken breast strips on a greased cookie sheet. Drizzle with olive oil mixture. Sprinkle spice mixture on top. You may need to turn the strips over to put some of the spice mix on the other side also.

Bake at 400 F for 18-20 minutes or until internal temperature of the chicken reaches 160 F.

Kale salad

Ingredients

Creamy Lemon Tahini Dressing

3 tablespoons tahini

3 tablespoons fresh lemon juice

1 tablespoon maple syrup or raw honey

1 tablespoon tamari (gluten-free soy sauce)

1/2 teaspoon turmeric

1 pinch crushed red pepper flakes

2 garlic cloves peeled and minced

1/4 cup olive oil extra virgin

Salad

1 bunch kale dino kale is best

1 cup purple cabbage shredded

1 cup carrots shredded

1/2 cup raw pumpkin seeds

1 avocado diced

1/4 cup hemp seeds shelled

1/4 cup goji berries or dried cranberries

Instructions

Whisk all dressing ingredients together in a bowl OR place them in a blender for 30 seconds until smooth. Taste and make adjustments to dressing, if necessary. Add a few tablespoons of filtered water to thin it out if needed. I like mine thick.

In a large bowl, place kale greens and add dressing. Massage dressing into kale leaves for about 2 minutes (until volume reduces by about 1/3). Add purple cabbage and toss to coat. Let sit for 15-30 minutes, so the dressing can continue breaking down the kale and cabbage.

When ready to serve, add in shredded carrots, pumpkin seeds, avocado, hemp seeds, and goji berries (if using). Toss to combine.

SUPER SOUP

INGREDIENTS

3 stalks bok choy

2 cups baby carrots, peeled

4 cups mixed greens, kale, spinach, collard greens

1 onion, chopped

4 cloves garlic, minced

2 cups baby broccoli

2 cups butternut squash, chopped into cubes

2 red or orange peppers, chopped

1 tablespoon smoked paprika

1 teaspoon tumeric

2 teaspoon sea salt

1 tablespoon granulated garlic

1 teaspoon black pepper

1 juice of 1 lemon

64 oz organic vegetable broth

2 tablespoon fresh parsley for garnish

2 tablespoon pomegranate seeds

INSTRUCTIONS

Add all prepared vegetables to Instant Pot.* (Stove top instructions below.) I like my vegetable soup chunky, so my vegetables are not chopped small. If you prefer, you can chop your vegetables.

Add spices and lemon juice. Add vegetable broth, making sure that your liquid does not go over the maximum line in the inner pot.

Set Instant Pot for 8 minutes to pressure cook. After cooking is complete, let pressure release naturally NR for 10 minutes. Release pressure and remove lid when valve goes down.

Transfer soup to large serving bowl and dish out into individual serving bowls. Garnish with parsley and pomegranate seeds.

Simple Cod with Sauteed Spinach

Ingredients

For the Cod

2 tablespoons olive oil

2) 5 ounce cod filets

ground black pepper {or seasoning of your choice}

For the Spinach

1 tablespoon olive oil

2 cloves fresh garlic, minced

10 ounces fresh baby spinach

sea salt and pepper, to taste

1 wedge lemon juice, squeezed

Instructions

Heat the olive oil in a large skillet over medium heat. Season the cod with ground black pepper {or seasoning of your choice} and place it in the skillet. Sear the first side and flip over. Cover and cook for 4 to 5 minutes. Remove from pan and set aside.

Clean out the skillet and add olive oil. When oil is heated, add the garlic. Cook for one minute, stirring to keep it from burning.

Add a handful of spinach and toss to combine. Saute and stir until spinach is wilted.

Add another handful of spinach, wilt, and continue until all of the spinach is wilted. Squeeze one wedge of lemon over the spinach and toss to combine. Season to taste with sea salt and pepper.

Divide the spinach between two plates, using a slotted spoon to drain off excess moisture. Top with the cod and season with black pepper and lemon strips and serve.

Fodmap Chicken & Fresh Herb Paella

Ingredients

5 Boneless, skin on Chicken Thighs

2 tablespoons Garlic infused olive oil

2 cups (400 grams) Paella Rice

4 cups (1 liter) low fodmap friendly chicken or vegetable stock

1 teaspoon Smoked Paprika

4-5 threads Saffron

1 teaspoon Sea Salt

1/2 teaspoon Black Pepper

1 Lemon Zest and Juice

1 cup (150 grams) Peas

1 bunch Spring Onions, (green part only) chopped

small handful about 1/3 cup of 10 g Fresh Parsley chopped

small handful about 1/3 cup of 10 g Fresh Mint chopped

small handful about 1/3 cup of 10 g Fresh Dill chopped

Need help converting to weights? Check out my cups to grams Conversion Guide.

Instructions

Place the chicken thighs on a cutting board and sprinkle with a generous amount of salt and pepper on both sides.

Warm a large pan/skillet over a medium-high heat. Add the garlic infused olive oil.

Add the chicken, skin-side down in the hot pan. Let the chicken cook, undisturbed for about 10 minutes or until the skin is golden brown.

Once the skin side is crispy and golden flip over and cook the other side, an addition 5-10 minutes until fully cooked. Once cooked through, transfer to clean plate and set aside for later. Wipe down the pan removing any remaining burnt bits and excess oil. Set the pan aside as well.

Rice prep: place the paella in a large pot and cover with stock. Add the lemon zest, half of the lemon juice, paprika, saffron, salt, and pepper. Bring the the pot to a simmer over a medium heat and let cook 15-20 minutes. Stir every so often.

Stir the peas and remaining half of the lemon juice in to the rice.

Transfer the rice to the skillet used to cook the chicken in along with the chopped herbs. Place the chicken back in the skillet with the rice and leave on the lowest heat setting and allow everything to rest for a couple of minutes before serving.

BARLEY SOUP RECIPE

Ingredients

¾ cup pearl barley

pieces1 celery stalk diced into small

1 onion diced into small pieces

1-2 medium carrot peeled and diced into small pieces

1 tomato diced into small pieces

2-3 cloves garlic finely chopped

3 cups chicken broth (or vegetable broth if vegan)

2 cups water

1 teaspoon finely chopped ginger

¼ cup chopped spring onions

1 tablespoon cooking oil

1 teaspoon dried thyme

salt and pepper

Instructions

Heat oil in a large pot over medium heat. Add ginger, garlic and saute until fragrant for about 30-40 sec

Add onions and saute until lightly golden brown for about a min. or two

Then add all the remaining ingredients except spring onions and let it boil.

Simmer on low heat for about 30 min. or until the barley is tender

Garnish with spring onions and serve warm to enjoy a bowl of barley soup

Cabbage Soup

Ingredients

garlic

onions

cabbage

canned tomatoes

chicken broth

1 tablespoon olive oil

1 white onion diced

3 cloves garlic minced

1/2 small head green cabbage chopped

2 cups slivered carrots

1 red bell pepper diced (optional)

14 ounces can diced tomatoes with spices

4 cups strong chicken broth

Instructions

In a large stockpot, fry the onions in the olive oil until soft. Add in the garlic and sautee until light brown.

Add in the rest of the vegetables, the tomatoes and the broth.

Simmer until the vegetables are soft , around 40-50 minutes, then serve.

EASY TURMERIC CHICKEN

INGREDIENTS

2 teaspoons extra-virgin olive oil

1 1/2 lbs. boneless, skinless chicken breasts, cut in about 1/2 inch cubes

1 1/4 teaspoons turmeric

3/4 teaspoon ground cumin

3/4 teaspoon kosher salt

1/4 teaspoon black pepper

1/8 teaspoon cayenne pepper (optional)

Juice of 1/2 lemon

INSTRUCTIONS

Heat a large skillet over medium heat and add olive oil.

Season chicken pieces with turmeric, cumin, salt, pepper and cayenne, if using.

Add chicken to the pan and cook until cooked through, 8-10 minutes, stirring occasionally.

Squeeze lemon juice over cooked chicken, serve warm and enjoy!

Anti- inflammatory juice

INGREDIENTS

4 celery stalks

½ cucumber

1 cup pineapple

½ green apple

1 cup spinach

1 lemon

1 knob ginger

INSTRUCTIONS

Add all ingredients to vegetable juicer.

Gently stir juice and consume immediately.

Conclusion

The conclusion of "Taming Gastritis: A Flavorful Journey to Digestive Wellness Cookbook" emphasizes the importance of managing gastritis through a balanced and nutritious diet. It summarizes the key takeaways and highlights the most effective dietary strategies to reduce inflammation and promote gut healing.

The conclusion stresses that the cookbook is not a substitute for medical advice or treatment, but rather a complementary tool to help manage symptoms and promote long-term digestive health. It encourages readers to work with their healthcare providers to develop a comprehensive treatment plan that incorporates both diet and other interventions.

The conclusion also emphasizes the importance of self-care and mindful eating, and provides practical tips for incorporating these practices into daily life. It encourages readers to listen to their bodies, honor their hunger and fullness cues, and savor the delicious and nutritious meals that can be prepared using the recipes in the book.

Ultimately, the conclusion of "Taming Gastritis" encourages readers to take an active role in their own health and wellness, and provides them with the tools and information they need to make informed decisions about their dietary choices and habits